How to Flatten Your Stomach

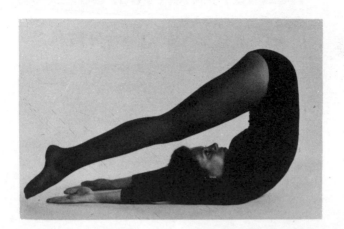

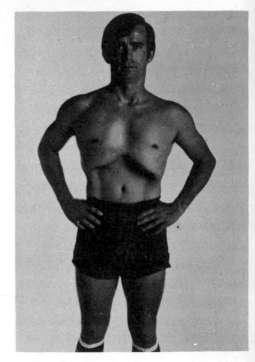

Coach Jim Everroad

How to Flatten Your Stomach

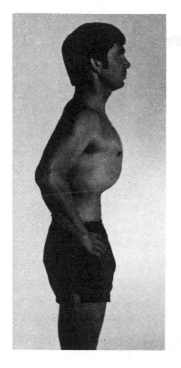

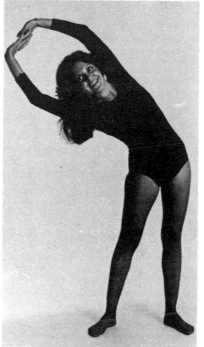

Pan Books

First published in America by Price/Stern/Sloan Publishers, Inc
410 North La Cienega Boulevard,
Los Angeles, California 90048
First published in Great Britain 1979 by Pan Books Ltd,
Cavaye Place, London SW10 9PG
© James M. Everroad 1974, 1975, 1978
ISBN 0 330 25877 X
Printed and bound in Great Britain by
Hazell Watson & Viney Ltd, Aylesbury, Bucks

Contents

Acknowledgements

The encouragement, cooperation, and enthusiasm of many people has led to the completion of this book. Thanks to all who have helped. Special thanks to Mr John Bare, Mr Al Gruber, Mrs Dottie Kinney, Mr Marty Shahbaz, and Miss Jan Young.

Thanks also to the *Gary Post Tribune* for the use of their photographs in the original edition.

Preface

Since I first published this book, the enormous interest in flat stomachs has come as a source of surprise and satisfaction to me. An even greater satisfaction has been the response I've received from people who use this programme. I've received letters and phone calls from people who are excited about their success, and multiple re-orders from others who have interested their friends in the programme.

The positive effects of exercise on muscle strength have been known for centuries. To achieve your flat stomach, you need only apply the proper exercises to the abdominal muscles. There are a large number of exercises in the programme for three reasons. One, different movements strengthen different muscle fibres, and the more different movements you perform, the more muscle fibres you'll strengthen. Two, it gets boring doing the same exercises every day. A large number of exercises will keep you interested in the programme. Three, you might not be able to do some of the exercises at first, and the easier ones will help condition you for the harder ones. In this book I have described the best exercises I've found for the abdominals.

My credentials include fifteen years as an athlete, ten more years as a high school gymnastics coach, and at least twenty years as a highly potential pot-belly prospect.

J. Everroad

Why flatten your stomach?

Appearance

'Looks' are a principal reason for flattening your stomach. Looks are important because the way you look helps to determine your self-image, and therefore the way you behave. A better self-image will help you act in such a manner as to better satisfy your desires. If you think you look better, you're more likely to make yourself happier. Also, the way you look helps to determine how people respond to you, and you to them.

The reactions of people to you helps you to decide several things. One, how you *want* to respond to them. Two, how you *can* respond to them. Three, how you *will* respond to them. Ultimately, then, the success or failure of your relationships is to some degree decided by your looks.

Your personal happiness and the success of your interpersonal relationships do, of course, depend on many things. Your concern with these things is obviously important. But it is equally obvious that your concern for your appearance is reasonable and important. There are many ways that you, or anyone, can improve on nature; and one of these is to flatten your stomach. There is another reason for this programme, which you may consider more important.

Health

Anatomy and physiology

The muscles which this programme is designed to strengthen are important for maintaining your health. They are the external obliques, internal obliques, rectus abdominus, and transversus abdominus. They attach to the middle of your chest, your lower eight ribs, your hip bones, the pelvis, to a line down the middle of your stomach, to tissues in your lower back, and to ligaments which are attached to your pelvis. The fibres of these muscles run in different directions, making them capable of great strength. Unfortunately, few people in our society perform the many different movements needed to tone these muscles.

It is important also to strengthen the muscles which work in direct opposition to the abdominal muscles. The most important of these opposing muscles is the diaphragm. The diaphragm is a large sheet of muscle which forms the entire roof, and part of the sides, of the abdominal cavity. Also, the erector spinae and the quadratus lumborum in the back, and the external intercostals in the rib cage, provide some opposition to the abdominals.

The abdominals, with the diaphragm, form most of the walls of the largest of your body's cavities. This cavity,

The abdomino-pelvic, extends from high under your rib cage to the floor of your pelvic bone. There are a number of organs here, which provide many life sustaining functions. Two important ways these muscles aid your health are by supporting and protecting these organs.

The abdomino-pelvic organs include the liver, gall bladder, stomach, small and large intestines, pancreas, spleen, bladder, kidneys, suprarenal glands and the sex organs. Their physiological functions include at least: digestion; production and storage of bile; formation of pancreatic juice and insulin; metabolism of lipids, carbohydrates and proteins; and storage of amino acids, iron and vitamins. Lymph is also formed; your body's acid base and water balances are maintained; blood is cleansed of waste products; the hormones of several endocrine glands are produced and emptied into the blood stream; also, plasma proteins and anti-bodies are produced. The abdomino-pelvic organs have many other functions, but these are enough to show the importance of their proper support and protection. If your abdominal muscles become stronger, it will be harder for a blow to your abdomen to damage these organs.

Sheets of tissue, called the peritoneum and fibrous membranes, keep these organs in place. These membranes contain elastic tissue, which is capable of considerable distention. Strong abdominal muscles lend much support to these membranes, thus helping to contain the organs.

These organs work according to chemical and

mechanical laws. A badly distended abdomen would probably not affect their chemical actions, but such distension could inhibit their mechanical workings, resulting in inefficiency.

Direct functions

The action of the abdominals and their opposing muscles causes pressure in the abdomino-pelvic cavity to increase and decrease. Because of this, they act directly in breathing, elimination of wastes, vomiting and in childbirth.

This programme is not designed for use by pregnant women, although its use beyond pregnancy is certainly worthwhile. If a woman's musculature is strong prior to pregnancy, she will have less difficulty carrying her baby and may have less difficulty in childbirth. Use of the programme after pregnancy will definitely help in restrengthening her abdominal muscles.

During vomiting, there is a strong, sudden contraction of the abdominals and the diaphragm. The contraction of the diaphragm causes it to move down on to the abdominal cavity, thereby increasing internal pressure. The internal pressure of the cavity is further increased as the abdominals tighten, decreasing its size. When the cavity pressure increases dramatically and suddenly, vomiting results. Without sufficient muscular strength, the act of vomiting becomes more difficult.

The action of the abdominal muscles generally aids the contraction of the walls of the rectum when solid wastes are eliminated. If you become constipated from having missed one or two bowel movements, the action of the abdominals becomes more important. If the internal pressure doesn't increase enough, the constipating waste will remain. If the internal pressure does increase enough, this waste will be eliminated. Obviously, the stronger the abdominals and the diaphragm, the more internal pressure can be generated. It is easier, then, to become constipated and harder to overcome this problem, if the abdominal muscles are weak.

A word of warning. In the event of constipation, people often attempt to increase the abdomino-pelvic pressure considerably. This 'straining' should be avoided if the constipation is chronic or the result of some ailment; your doctor should be consulted.

A further warning. Normally, if a person is 'pot bellied', his abdominal muscles are weak. This same person may have a strong diaphragm. These two statements are true because: (1) few people receive more than minimal abdominal exercise; (2) everyone exercises their diaphragm continuously while breathing. If such a person strains during constipation, the weak abdominal wall will yield to pressure generated by the descending diaphragm. This could cause pain and possibly the common inguinal hernia, in the weakest areas of the abdominal wall. If you are an older athlete who has neglected his or her stomach, although being involved in a heavy fitness programme, take heed.

A final warning about bowel habits. The uses of laxatives or enemas are abused by many people. Over-use or dependence on them can lead to problems with the digestive tract, such as irritable or inactive colon. People with misconceptions about bowel habits may imagine they are constipated when they are not. This imaginary constipation can lead to real problems, if the bowels are improperly stimulated by laxatives or enemas. Again, if you have questions about this, see your doctor. Strengthening your abdominal muscles can aid bowel habits, thus helping you avoid laxative misuse.

The abdominals also help support the lower part of your backbone. Lower back pain is a common problem in people over forty. If you wish to prevent this problem, exercising the muscles of the lower back and stomach will help. This programme does exercise both areas. Also, if you currently suffer from lower back pain, the programme could be useful as therapy. Since the pain could have causes besides muscular weakness, you should talk to your doctor.

Over-eating

An important reason for abdominal strength, which concerns both your appearance and your health, is its effect on over-eating. People who are overweight tend to eat until they feel full. Higher internal abdomino-pelvic pressure results from increased abdominal strength. This increased pressure will cause you to feel fullness sooner than when the abdominals are weak. This feeling of fullness can make you stop eating sooner, keeping you from stuffing yourself. You may, of course, decide to stuff yourself anyhow. But the stronger the muscles become, the easier it will be to pay attention to 'fullness', and the more uncomfortable it will be to stuff your stomach. With no conscious effort towards dieting, you could build the strength to cause a reduction in food intake. Reducing food intake can yield many pleasant results.

Over-eating is one cause of many problems. Some of the common ones are indigestion, heartburn, and diarrhoea. Increased abdominal strength will help you avoid these problems, and others.

Well, maybe you consider your looks, rather than your health, the more important reason to flatten your stomach. But I hope you realize that improved abdominal strength will help you improve and maintain your health.

Obesity

A word about obesity. Most people know that obesity is associated with an enormous number of health problems, which include heart and circulatory diseases, lower back pain and degenerative joint disease. If you carry too much body fat, you should eliminate as much as desirable. But remember that this programme is designed to strengthen muscles, not eliminate fat.

A good deal of dieting or of exercise is necessary to reduce a single kilogramme of body fat. The best reducing programmes include both exercise and diet. This one is an important supplement to any fat reduction programme. It can aid your diet by helping you lower your food intake, as I've explained. It will supplement many exercise programmes, because they fail to tone the abdominal wall sufficiently.

To understand obesity better, and to avoid being hoodwinked by thousands of diet fads, mechanical aids and other fat reduction programmes, you should read a book called *Overweight*. The book is written by Jean Mayer who is, in my opinion, probably the world's finest authority on the subject. You can find it at your local library. But if your problem is serious, it's worth buying. Ask a local bookshop to order it. It is published by Prentice-Hall.

Summary

There are, then, at least seven reasons for using this programme for flattening your stomach:

1. It will improve your appearance.

2. It will create better support and protection for your abdomino-pelvic organs.

3. It will help improve those functions in which the abdominal muscles act directly.

4. It will help you avoid the misuse of laxatives.

5. It will help you avoid problems such as hernias and lower back pain, and may be used in their therapy.

6. It will help you avoid over-eating, and other related health problems.

7. It is an important supplement to any fat reduction programme (diet and/or exercises), and any other exercise programme.

How to use this programme

Your goal is to build and maintain a flat stomach *easily*. This is going to take time. You will be doing a limited number of exercises, and limited repetitions of each exercise. Why? Because you will want to go on with an easy programme, and you'd probably give up a strenuous one. If you stay with this programme, it will definitely help. If you give up any programme, it won't work.

You may feel improved abdominal strength in a few weeks, or even in a few days. By all means be encouraged, but don't expect comments from others about your new physique. You probably won't *see* improved flatness in your stomach for a month or more. When your waist line starts to decrease (it will), and you can tell your stomach is flatter with your shirt on, you still might not see muscles rippling in your stomach.

If muscular definition is what you want, you will probably need to do one or all of three things. One, step up this programme considerably. Two, get into another exercise programme designed to burn off more calories. Three, diet. This programme, as it's designed, may or may not build you a 'washboard' stomach. It will, however, flatten your stomach, and that is certainly worth those benefits mentioned in the first part of this book.

As with any exercise programme, you should check with your doctor. When you tell him that you're planning to go slowly, and that your goal is to flatten your stomach, he should be delighted. Later, when he sees you've been successful, he'll probably start the programme himself. The older you are, and the less you've been taking exercise, the more important this medical consultation becomes.

A word of caution. It might be a good idea not to tell anyone that you're going on this programme, especially your spouse, family or close friends. Exercise by anyone not actively engaged in an organized sport is so unusual in our sedentary society that people will probably think you're a 'ding-dong'. They'll discourage you with laughter and jokes, because of jealousy, or for almost any other reason. If your self-image is like mine (and like most people's), it won't stand up under too much criticism. Letting others know what you're doing could cause you to fail. Six months from now, when someone comments about the weight you've lost or how much better you look, do them a favour and tell them what you've been doing. They can't and won't argue with success. In fact they'll probably be proud of your initiative and efforts. It should be easy to talk them into trying your programme, instead of them talking you out of it.

Okay, let's get started. Begin by finding a time and place that you can be alone to do your exercises. You'll need very little time or space, so this shouldn't be difficult. The best time is usually in the morning when you first get up. Early exercisers are least likely to become drop-outs, although any time that's convenient is fine.

Measure your girth at the level of your navel with your stomach normally relaxed. Pull your stomach in as far as you can and measure it again. Record both measurements. Do this once a month on the same date each month. This is an effective means of recording your progress. A year from your first measurement, please drop me a note and let me know how you've done.

A good start for the first day would be two repetitions of the first ten exercises. It will take some time to *study* the descriptions of the exercises, and it is important to do them correctly. The second day you would do two repetitions of the second ten exercises. The first few days it is best to become familiar with the programme while doing little actual exercise. If you're excited and want to do more repetitions, it's up to you. But keep these two principles in mind: (1) unless you're working in a hot area, you shouldn't work up a sweat; (2) if you feel stiff or sore tomorrow, you did too much today. The exact amount of exercising you start with depends on your age and your physical condition. If you're an eighty-year-old retired 'desk jockey', you'll probably have to start lower and proceed more slowly than a thirty-year-old construction worker.

As you progress in the programme, you should lower the number of exercises per work-out, and increase the number of repetitions per exercise. For example, start with two repetitions of the first ten. The next work-out do two repetitions of the second ten. When you feel you can progress *easily,* begin doing three repetitions of the first eight in one work-out, three of the second eight in the next work-out, then three of the last four plus three of the first four in the third work-out. Continue rotating through the different exercises in the programme, doing three repetitions of eight different exercises in every work-out.

For the next increase you might do five times each of six exercises in a work-out, and six different exercises in each succeeding work-out, until you're ready for another increase. Then do seven repetitions of five exercises per work-out. Then ten of four exercises should be done. When you're finally up to doing four exercises a dozen times each, you begin to progress by adding a dozen repetitions of an additional exercise to your work-outs.

Unless you want to become an abdominal culturist, there is no reason to ever do more than a dozen repetitions of ten exercises per workout. And you should progress to this level only if it's easy, and only after much time in the programme. My current level is eight exercises each twelve times. I may progress further, and I may not.

If you become stiff or sore after the first, or any other day, there are several methods of relief:

1. Expose the stiffness or soreness to warm water. You can do this in a bath or shower.

2. Massage the stiff or sore area. This helps, especially if done in the bath or under the shower.

3. Reduce either the number of exercises in your work-outs or the number of repetitions per exercise, or both.

4. If a specific exercise seems too difficult or causes pain, soreness or stiffness, leave it out. After several months of conditioning, see if you can add it without strain. If not, leave it out again.

These exercises range from very simple to rather difficult. If you can do them all, fine. If not, do those which you can, and don't worry about the rest.

Start easy and stay easy.
Take plenty of time to achieve your goals.

This may seem difficult, but patience and persistence will reap many benefits. If your programme is easy enough, you'll stay with it permanently, and you'll keep your flat stomach for good!

Stomach flattening exercises

1 If you haven't read why you should flatten your stomach, or how to use this programme, go back and read that information first. Those sections contain information which you should know, and much of that material is essential to your success in the programme.

2 Stand with your back 30–60 cm (12–24 in) from a wall, feet shoulder-width apart, arms stretched overhead, elbows straight. Bend back and touch the wall with the fingernails, knees and elbows straight as possible (pictured). Return to starting position, and immediately bend forward and touch the floor, knees still as straight as possible. Return to starting position for one repetition.

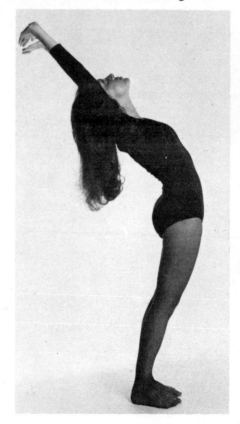

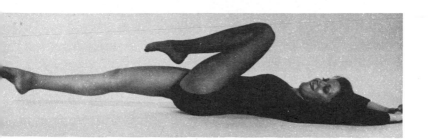

3 Lie on your back, arms stretched overhead against the floor, buttocks resting on the floor, feet off the floor and knees *drawn up close to the chest.* Extend one leg straight out, parallel to the floor, but not quite touching it (pictured). Draw the first knee back close to the chest, at the same time extending the second leg straight out. Draw the second knee back, while again extending the first leg, and continue this bicycling movement. Allow four extensions for one repetition of the exercise.

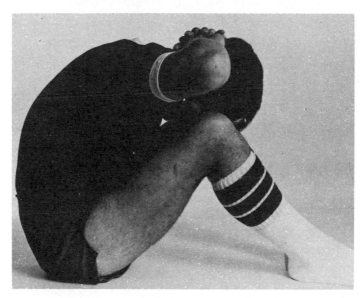

4 Lie on your back, legs bent, with the knees pointed at the ceiling, feet flat on the floor, hands on the back of your head, fingers interlocked. Exhale as you rise up, and place the head between the knees (pictured p27). Inhale as you lower back to starting position. It may help to place your feet under a piece of heavy furniture, such as a dresser or couch, or anything which helps to keep them in place.

5 It is possible to expand your chest after completely exhaling, in the same manner that your chest expands as you inhale. It is important to learn to do this, so that you can do properly both this exercise and exercise number 13. You have spent your entire life expanding your chest while inhaling, and relaxing it (allowing it to become smaller) while exhaling. Therefore, it will probably take some practice to be able to expand it after completely exhaling.

To practise, first inhale deeply, and try to consciously feel the way your chest expands. Next, think only of expanding your chest, and not of pulling in the air; just allow the air to come in as you expand your chest. You will find that you can expand your chest just as much when the air doesn't rush into your lungs. Finally, exhale completely, hold the exhalation, and expand your chest as you've learned to do. When you do this correctly, your stomach will automatically pull in deeply. Learning this action may take patience and practice, but it is well worth the effort! When you do this action properly, you are ready to do the exercise.

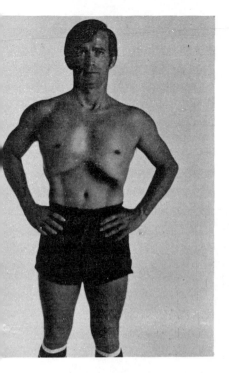
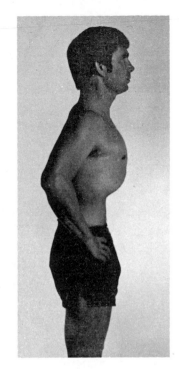

Stand, feet shoulder-width apart, hands on hips. Exhale completely and forcefully! Holding the exhalation, expand the chest as much as possible. Pull the stomach in tightly, and hold for up to 6 seconds (pictured). Relax to starting position. Do this exercise in front of a mirror to build confidence in your progress.

6 Stand, feet comfortably more than shoulder-width apart, arms stretched sideways and parallel to the floor, elbows straight. Keep the feet planted firmly on the ground, and slowly twist the trunk as far to the right as possible (pictured). Stretch, pulling the right arm back, and the left arm around to the right. Snap back to starting position, and place the hands on the hips. Return to starting position, and repeat to the left. Turning to right and then to left constitutes one repeat of the exercise.

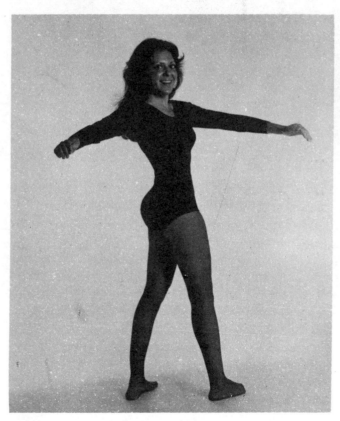

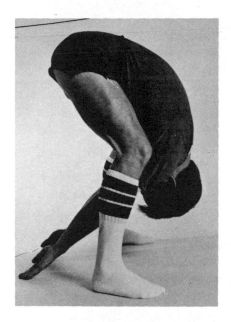

7 Stand, feet straddled as wide as comfortable, arms
overhead, elbows straight, hands shoulder-width apart.
Rapidly swing your upper body forward and down, *while
bending your knees.* Reach back through the legs and
touch the ground as far back as possible (pictured).
Swing the upper body back and stop suddenly, 'jerking'
to a stop at the starting position.

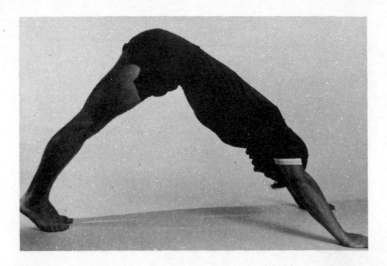

8 Lie on your stomach, hands above the hips and close to your sides, elbows pointed at the ceiling, palms on the floor with fingers pointed towards the shoulders. Keep the feet on the ground and raise the head, shoulders and chest as high as possible, arching the back. Keeping the hands and feet in place, lift the rear high, so that your body describes an upside-down V shape. Bearing the weight on the hands and feet, with knees and elbows straight, and remaining in the V, pull in the stomach and tighten it. Hold this position (pictured) for up to 6 seconds. Lower the rear to the original arched position, then back to starting position.

9 Sit, legs bent, knees pointed at the ceiling, feet flat on the floor (preferably supported under a piece of heavy furniture such as a dresser or a couch, or anything which helps to keep them in place, as in exercise 4), hands on the back of the head, fingers interlocked.

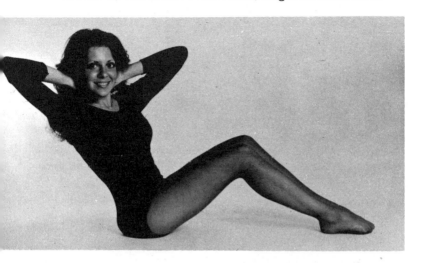

Lean back until your upper body is at a 45° angle, twist completely left, then right (pictured), then return forward and back to starting position (sitting). Twist to the left first on the first half of your repeats, then to the right first on the second half of your repeats.

10 Stand, feet shoulder-width apart, hands on hips. Reach over the top of the head with the left hand, touching the right ear. Bend over sideways to the right, sliding the right hand as far as possible down the right leg and stretching the left side as much as possible (pictured). Do not allow yourself to reach forwards or backwards in order to reach farther down with the right hand. Bend up to starting position and repeat to the left.

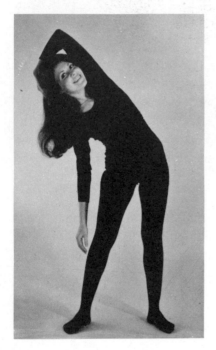

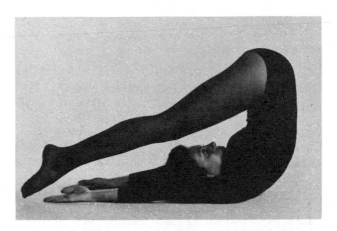

11 Lie on your back, legs straight and together, arms stretched overhead against the floor. Attempting to keep the legs straight, lift them up and over the head, continuing back and downwards, and trying to touch the floor with your toes (pictured). Return the legs through the same path to the starting position.

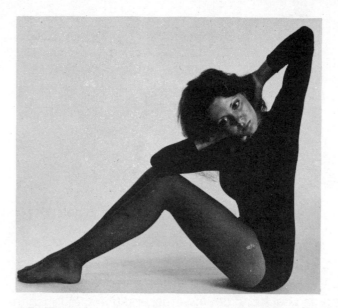

12 This exercise is the same as number 4, except that as you rise you twist the trunk and place the right elbow outside the left knee (pictured). Return to starting position. Twist to place the left elbow outside the right knee on the second half of your repeats of the exercise. Example: if you are doing it ten times, you twist to the left for the first five, then to the right for the second five. Do the repetitions on one side consecutively before doing them on the other side.

13 The ability to expand your chest after exhaling, as you did in exercise 5, is necessary for this exercise. Stand, bent at the waist and slightly at the knees, leaning forward to support the upper body-weight with the hands on the knees, elbows straight. Exhale completely and forcefully! Holding the exhalation, expand the chest as in exercise 5. Then push the stomach out, still holding the exhalation and chest expansion. A ridge of muscle (the rectus abdominus) should form between the rib cage and the pelvis (pictured). Tighten this ridge of muscle, and hold for up to 6 seconds. If you can't get the ridge to form at first, be patient and practise. After you've increased your repeats, it's a good idea to alternate repeats of exercise 5 with this one.

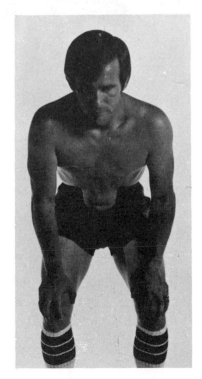

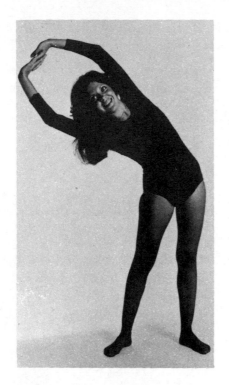

14 Stand, feet comfortably more than shoulder-width apart, arms straight overhead, elbows straight, palms towards ceiling, with fingers interlocked. Bend sideways to the right as far as possible, stretching the left side (pictured). Straighten and bend immediately back, stretching the arms and shoulders backwards. Straighten and bend forwards, touching or nearly touching the palms on the floor. Return to starting position. Keep the knees straight throughout the exercise. Change directions, bending to the left after the first half of your repeats.

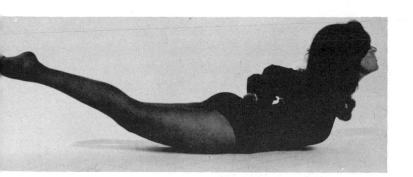

15 Lie on your stomach, hands clasped in the small of your back, legs straight. Raise the head, chest and shoulders as high as possible, at the same time raising the feet and legs, also to their maximum (pictured). Hold momentarily, then lower to starting position.

16 Stand, feet shoulder-width apart, arms at sides, elbows straight. Lift your right hip sideways towards your right shoulder, allowing your right foot to come off the ground. *Don't* move the right leg sideways. Also don't think of lifting your right foot, just *allow* it to come up. Lift the hip high, trying to touch the hip and your lowest rib together (pictured). Return to the starting

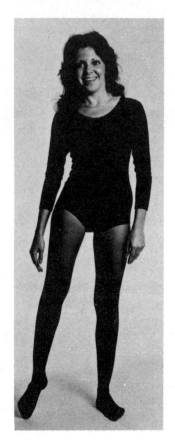

position, then repeat on the *same* side. The movement repeated twice in succession on the left side is also one repeat. Do the first half on one side, the second half on the other. Example: if you're doing ten repeats, you do five (ten successive hip lifts) on one side, then five on the other.

17 In the last part of this exercise, again it is necessary to have your chest expanded while your lungs are *exhaled,* as in exercises 5 and 13. This time you expand the chest to its maximum by *inhaling*; then, you keep the chest expanded as you exhale completely.
Practising this action may help you to learn the other exercises. To practise, inhale completely, then keep your chest expanded as you exhale. When you have the action right, your stomach will pull in deeply as you exhale. Then you are ready for one of this programme's finest exercises!

18 Stand straight, feet together, arms at your sides. Rotate your pelvis as the arrows in the picture indicate, then straighten your back, pulling the shoulders back. Without relaxing, again rotate the pelvis, then again straighten the back and shoulders. Without relaxing, repeat the action a third time. By now the chest will be held high and tremendously expanded, and your stomach will be pulled in deeply. Your back will be extremely straight and your shoulders far back. In this exaggerated position of attention, inhale forcefully, expanding the chest to its maximum. Hold for 6 counts. Without relaxing, exhale completely and forcefully, tighten your abdominals (pictured), and hold for 6 seconds. Relax to starting position.

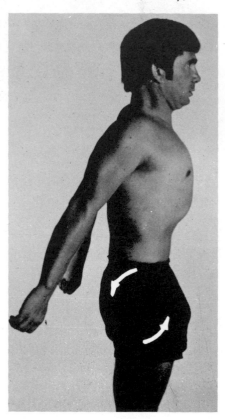

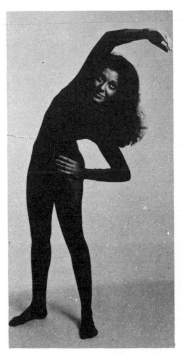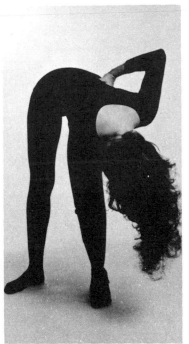

19 Stand, feet comfortably more than shoulder-width apart, hands on hips. Reach sideways, then straight overhead, with the right arm. Stretching the right side thoroughly, continue moving the right arm plus the upper body to the left and downwards. Remain stretched at the shoulder as long as you maintain the sideways motion, and keep the sideways motion as long as possible (left). Allow yourself to twist forwards at the waist at the end of the movement and, keeping the legs straight, attempt to touch the floor outside the left foot (right). Return through the same path to the starting position. Repeat the movement, with the left arm moving to the right, and relax.

20 Lie on your back, feet together, toes pointed, arms stretched overhead against the floor, elbows straight, hands shoulder-width apart. Raise your legs, keeping them straight, until they are vertical (pictured). Lower the legs slowly to starting position.

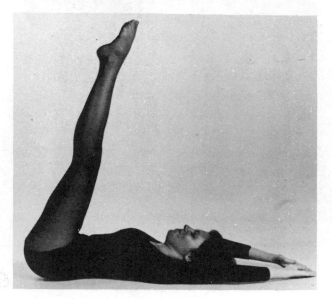

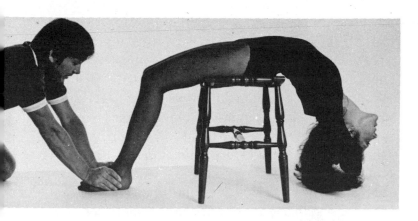

21 Sit in a chair, facing its back and straddling its back with your legs (use a stool if you have one available). The chair or stool should be 30–60 cm (1–2 ft) high, depending on your height and condition and what is available. Place your feet under a piece of heavy furniture as in exercise 4. Place the palms on top of the head, fingers interlocked. Lean back as far as you can, touching the interlocked fingers on the ground, if possible (pictured). Pull up through starting position while exhaling, and lean forwards as much as you can. Return to starting position.

This is one of the more difficult exercises. If you can perform it completely, you should make progress fairly rapidly. If you can't do the whole movement now, the day you do it will be an excellent mark of your progress.

22 Fasten a piece of thread around your waist at the level of your navel. Fasten it so it's 5–10 cm (2–4 in) smaller than your girth when you are normally relaxed. Pull your stomach in until your girth is as small as the circumference of the thread, and keep it pulled in to this size. Leave the thread there as long as possible, and at least for 4–5 hours. This is a great way to remind yourself, every time you relax your stomach, to tighten your abdominal muscles. Keep the thread there, especially when you are sitting and when you are eating. Using this technique you automatically begin the programmes with a 5–10 cm (2–4 in) smaller girth. This is not a trick but a legitimate form of exercise. Thread works best for this purpose because it's uncomfortable enough to keep you honest. Avoid using wide objects for this purpose, since you'll tend to use them instead of muscular effort to hold in your stomach.

The thread will tend to roll up and down your waist. To keep it in place, tape it to your skin at 6–8 points around your waist. This technique works best when you are wearing loose clothing.

Good luck with your programme. Work at it, and it will work for you. If you have questions concerning the programme, or if you wish to send me a progress report, address your correspondence to:

Coach Jim Everroad
2698 Wildwood Lane
Columbus, Indiana 47201
USA

Bruce Tulloh
The Complete Jogger £1

Jogging needs no skill, yet it's a certain way to improve your heart, looks, breathing and longevity – as well as controlling your weight. All you need is a little guidance from an experienced runner on how to start, and how to get maximum benefit from jogging schedules that suit your needs and lifestyle – the guidance given by one of Britain's best known runners, Bruce Tulloh, in this book.

Peter F. Drucker
The Effective Executive 95p

'A specific and practical book about how to be an executive who *contributes* . . .

The purpose of this book is to induce the executive to concentrate on his own contribution and performance, with his attention directed to improving the organization by serving outsiders better. I believe Mr Drucker achieves this purpose simply and brilliantly – and in the course of doing so offers many insights into executive work and suggestions for improving executive performance.

I can conscientiously recommend that this book be given the very highest priority for executive reading and even re-reading' DIRECTOR

Margaret Hennig and Anne Jardim
The Managerial Woman 90p

'Why do so many women founder on the lowly rungs of the executive ladder? *The Managerial Woman* attempts to provide an answer by telling ambitious women how to overcome the worst pitfalls' DAILY MAIL

'For this book 3,000 women were involved in seminars or interviews and 25 who had made it were interviewed in great depth' DIRECTOR

You can buy these and other Pan Books from booksellers and newsagents; or direct from the following address:
Pan Books, Sales Office, Cavaye Place, London SW10 9PG
Send purchase price plus 20p for the first book and 10p for each additional book, to allow for postage and packing
Prices quoted are applicable in the UK

While every effort is made to keep prices low, it is sometimes necessary to increase prices at short notice. Pan Books reserve the right to show on covers and charge new retail prices which may differ from those advertised in the text or elsewhere